EMERGENCY DENTISTRY HANDBOOK

EMERGENCY DENTISTRY HANDBOOK

Providing Dental Care in Disaster Areas, Combat Zones, and Other Austere Environments

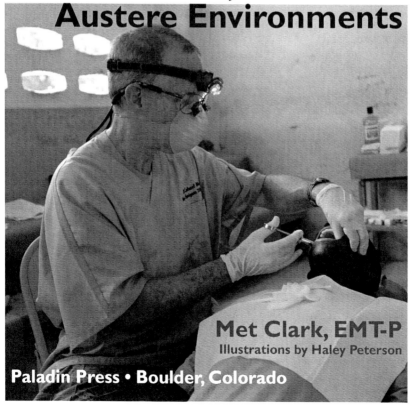

Met Clark, EMT-P

Illustrations by Haley Peterson

Paladin Press • Boulder, Colorado

Emergency Dentistry Handbook:
Providing Dental Care in Disaster Areas, Combat Zones,
and Other Austere Environments
by Met Clark, EMT-P

Copyright © 2011 by Met Clark

ISBN 13: 978-1-161004-044-0
Printed in the United States of America

Published by Paladin Press, a division of
Paladin Enterprises, Inc.
Gunbarrel Tech Center
7077 Winchester Circle
Boulder, Colorado 80301 USA
+1.303.443.7250

Direct inquiries and/or orders to the above address.

Cover photo: Air Force Lt. Col. Richard Moore, a dentist with 56th Medical Group,
prepares a local patient for a tooth extraction at the U.S. Army South New Horizons–
Haiti 2010 Ennery medical assistance site July 13. (Photo credit: Spc. Jessica M.
Lopez, Task Force Kout Men Public Affairs)

Visit our website at www.paladin-press.com

CONTENTS

WARNING

The techniques and procedures in this book are only to be administered by certified medical professionals. This book is not meant to be a substitute for proper and thorough education and training in the fields of medicine and emergency first aid.

The author, publisher, and distributors of this book disclaim any liability from any damages or injuries of any type that a reader or user of information contained in this book may encounter from the use or misuse of said information.

PREFACE

Emergency Dentistry Handbook is written for all levels of medical professionals who may find themselves in a remote and austere environment. The environments may range from assisting disaster areas in the United States to providing humanitarian aid in Afghanistan or missionary work in the Congo. No matter where the medical professional may find him or herself, the objective of this guide is to provide emergency dental information that will assist the medical operational platform. This guide is not intended to be a substitute for professional dental work, nor is the author, publisher, or distributors of this book liable for persons working outside of their scope of practice. The information contained within is intended to help bridge the gap until definitive care can be given by a trained dental professional.

Emergency Dentistry Handbook focuses on operations in remote areas around the world, and its recommendations for treatment of injuries and diseases reflect this. It strives to offer a base template and recognizes the fact that several methodologies and treatments are available, while others may be unavailable under difficult and primitive conditions. It is the responsibility of the medical practitioner/operator to stay up to date on new trends and appropriate pharmaceutical literature and remain flexible when various treatment options are not available due to regional, cultural, or tribal circumstances.

The first rule of medicine applies, no matter the circumstance or area of operation: DO NO HARM.

INTRODUCTION

Emergency dentistry skills are valuable tools to any organization. Armed conflict, disaster relief, missionary work, and humanitarian aid are examples of situations where a medical professional may come into contact with a patient experiencing dental pain under adverse conditions. In these environments, a properly trained medical practitioner/operator can provide dental services in forward areas of operation, assist dental officers, and identify dental emergencies that require evacuation to a higher level of care.

Treating the patient with simple dental first aid may be all that is required. Most dental emergencies are seldom life threatening, but the pain can be so severe that the patient becomes incapacitated and demoralized. Managing dental pain will vary between different practitioners, but it mainly consists of prescribing an antibiotic regimen, administering pain medication, or, as a last resort, extracting the offending tooth.

GOALS FOR AUSTERE AND EMERGENCY DENTISTRY

❏ Check airway, breathing, and circulation (ABCs) first!
❏ Give thorough examination.
❏ Manage pain.
❏ Treat appropriately.
❏ Refer to definitive care.
❏ Keep accurate documentation.

1. Always check the ABCs. Maxillofacial trauma may occlude the patient's airway and present life-threatening injuries that must be addressed first. Continue with dental care after the concerns of the ABCs have been met. Many dental injuries can be treated with simple dental first aid.
2. Conduct a thorough examination of all the surrounding tissues and bones for injuries, diseases, infections, foreign bodies, and missing teeth.
3. Manage the patient's pain. If you are unable to provide total pain relief, then make the pain tolerable for the patient. Use the appropriate pain-management protocol that will provide the best relief, while allowing for healing and evacuation time. Streamline the dental care for simplicity and sustainment of continual support.
4. Treat appropriately within your scope of practice. If you are trained in dental first aid, then apply dental first aid. Do not use treatments and procedures that you are not trained in. Your objective is to provide temporary relief until a higher level of professional dental care can be given.
5. Refer to definitive care. Some dental injuries are true emergencies, and the best care for the patient is to be seen by a dental specialist in the shortest possible time frame. Limited and restricted access due to remote locations, disaster environments, operational sensitivity, or austere settings will delay evacuation of the patient. It is imperative to have an operational dental plan that encompasses training, predeployment and deployment examinations, emergency evacuations, and follow-up care.
6. Provide accurate documentation of all dental injuries, diseases, infections, and missing teeth. Use diagrams, drawings, and charts to identify the location of the injuries and treatments given.

PREVENTIVE DENTISTRY

Preventive dentistry is a very important component of emergency dentistry. Many of the complications associated with toothaches can be avoided with simple brushing and flossing techniques. Medical practitioners/operators deployed into disaster, humanitarian, missionary, and combat environments must not only maintain proper oral fitness themselves; they also must provide education and training programs for their fellow operators, health-care providers, soldiers, and relief workers. Maintaining proper oral hygiene increases morale and will help sustain the operational tempo in deployed environments. Dental pain and injuries can be incapacitating, but most problems are easily treated with dental first aid.

Another aspect of preventive maintenance for soldiers and health=care workers deployed in a remote setting is the ability to educate the local populace in proper oral care. An educational outreach program will help foster good relations through distribution of toothbrushes, toothpaste, and dental floss. Educate the local populace by placing emphasis on proper diet and nutrition. Most caries (decaying and crumbling of a tooth) can be prevented by simply reducing the amount of refined sugar consumed in food and beverages. Effective educational programs will help lessen the workload of seeing patients at the clinic in current, ongoing, and future operations.

ANATOMY

The structures of the oral cavity consist of the lips, the tongue, the inner/outer cheeks, and the floor and roof of the mouth, including the soft and hard palate.

The maxilla and the mandible make up the upper and lower jaw. Teeth fit into sockets, called the alveoli, in the jaw and are held in place along the alveolar ridge. Each socket is composed of the periodontal ligament, the bone socket, and the gingiva, or gum. The gingiva should always feel firm to the touch and fit closely around the tooth. Bleeding along the gingiva should be noted for disease processes that can be controlled with proper oral hygiene.

In the first two years of human development, 20 teeth are formed and are called the primary or deciduous teeth. These teeth form two rows of 10 on the upper jaw and 10 on the lower jaw. The teeth are further broken down into four front teeth, known as the incisors, two canines, and four molars for each jawline.

Permanent teeth begin to emerge and replace the primary teeth between the ages of 6 and 12. By the time adulthood is reached, 32 permanent teeth should be formed, broken down into two rows of 16 teeth. The teeth are the four front teeth (incisors), two canines, four premolars, and six molars. The third molar, or wisdom tooth, typically erupts in early adulthood.

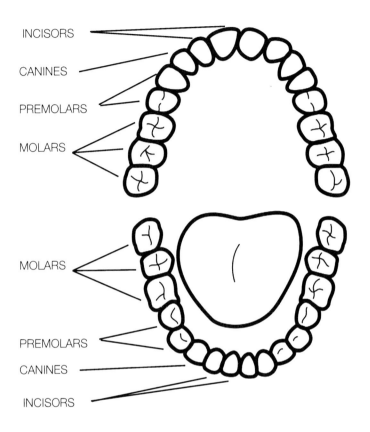

INCISORS

CANINES

PREMOLARS

MOLARS

MOLARS

PREMOLARS

CANINES

INCISORS

The incisors and canines have cutting edges that are intended for ripping and tearing. The premolars are transitional teeth between the canines and molars. The food is introduced to the canines and incisors for initial tearing and then passed along to the premolars. The premolars capture, tear, rip, and pregrind the food before it is passed along to the molars for final grinding.

Salivation ducts are located near the upper left and right molars on the mucosa membrane of the cheeks and behind the front teeth along the floor of the mouth.

The temporomandibular joint is the point of articulation, or hinge, between the upper and lower jaw. The temporomandibular joint is the common site for dislocation due to traumatic impact, yawning, or general weakening of the joint.

The tooth consists of two primary parts, called the crown and the root. The crown is the top portion of the tooth that is visible in the mouth. The root is embedded in the sockets of the alveoli and cannot be seen in the mouth. Trauma to the mouth can expose the root of the tooth.

The tooth has three layers. The outer portion, called the enamel or crystalline, is an extremely hard, mineralized surface that covers the crown. The second layer, called the dentin, is the core of the tooth. The third layer is the innermost portion of the tooth, called the pulp. The pulp chamber consists of the blood vessels and nerves that connect the tooth to the jaw at the apices of the tooth. The periodontal ligament attaches the root of the tooth to the alveolar bone.

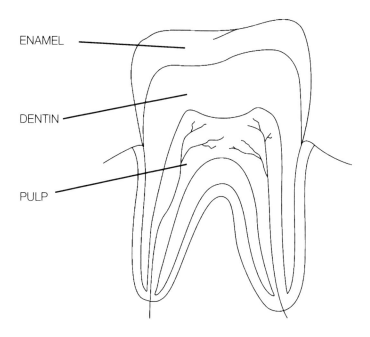

SURFACES OF THE TOOTH

For descriptive and documentation purposes, the following terms are useful:

- Occlusal surface—The chewing surface of the molars and pre-molars.
- Lingual surface—The surface closest to the tongue in the lower jaw and the palatal surface of the upper jaw (i.e., along the inside of the teeth).
- Buccal surface—The surface closest to the lips and cheeks (i.e., along the outside of the teeth).
- Mesial surface—The surface closest to the midline of the body.
- Distal surface—The surface farthest from the midline of the body.

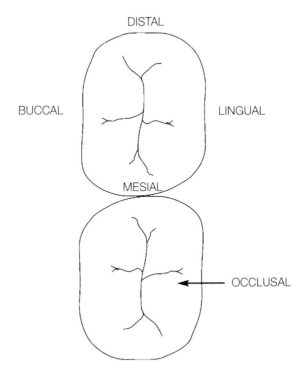

MEDICATIONS

The medications discussed in this chapter are merely recommendations for use in emergency dentistry care. The medical practitioner/operator will choose the appropriate medications based upon global availability, intent of use, and the dictates of local laws, regulations, and customs. The medications offered in the following guidelines are generally accepted globally.

It is the practitioner/operator's responsibility to record administration history and dosages in the patient's record. The practitioner/operator is personally responsible for staying up to date on current medication trends, including knowing proper dosages, routes of administration, and contraindications of use.

When using narcotics, refer to the appropriate dental protocol established by the organization or agency. The use of narcotics requires the practitioner/operator to adhere to strict protocol and control of the substance. Regional laws and tribal customs dictate serious repercussions if the practitioner/operator does not abide by protocol or maintain control of the substance during administration.

If the patient is on IV administration for medications, it is recommended to switch to oral administration when appropriate. Oral antibiotics, painkillers, and other medications will decrease the workload in remote areas, where patients must travel great distances to be seen by a medical practitioner/operator.

The Mallampati scale is helpful in determining when to move the patient from IV to oral administration. A Mallampati scale of 2 indicates an intercisal opening of 20mm, or the equivalent of two fingers. The Mallampati scale of 2 will serve as an evaluation tool for determining if the patient's mouth will be mobile enough to ingest oral medications. Other important considerations should include normal body temperature, no fluctuant areas at or near the afflicted site, and the patient's ability to eat a proper diet without difficulty.

PAIN MANAGEMENT

To manage dental pain in remote and austere environments, the administration of simple pain medications is the best practice. The practitioner/operator should make every attempt to avoid administering addictive pain medications to the patient; however, strong procedures that impede upon the nerves will require a stronger medical dosing.

The medical practitioner/operator may have a difficult time determining the level of pain that the patient is experiencing. Managing pain will be difficult, but it can be accomplished by adhering to the simple practice of making the patient feel comfortable and not overmedicated. The practitioner/operator will use heavier sedatives when the patient is unable to rest from the dental pain and procedures performed.

Below are common pain management medications, along with the most popular dosing. The practitioner/operator should also remain aware that pain management may be as simple as providing basic dental first aid or administering antibiotics for infections.

- Acetaminophen, 325–650 mg every 6 hours PO
- Ibuprofen, 400–800 mg every 6 hours PO
- Codeine, 60 mg every 4 hours PO as needed for pain
- Hydrocodone, 5 mg every 4-6 hours PO as needed for pain
- Morphine, 8-20 mg every 4 hours PO as needed for pain
- Oxycodone, 5 mg every 4-6 hours PO as needed for pain

ANTIBIOTICS

The typical administration period for antibiotics will last from 7 to 10 days. During this time frame, the patient must be advised to strictly adhere to the prescribed antibiotic regimen to maintain appropriate therapeutic levels. Administering antibiotics may be difficult to maintain due to limited available resources, harsh environment, local laws, tribal customs, or religious beliefs.

Penicillin

Penicillins are the most commonly prescribed antibiotic for oral infections. They inhibit bacterial cell wall synthesis. Use a loading dose to rapidly achieve therapeutic blood levels. Contraindications include allergies/sensitivities and poor renal function.

Penicillins are broken into four categorical spectrums: narrow, moderate, broad, and extended. Each category of penicillin will be more active against a susceptible organism.

REMEMBER! Always monitor the patient for sensitivity to penicillins during treatment for infections.

Pen VK and Pen G

Pen VK is commonly prescribed because of its solubility and oral administration properties. Other penicillins, such as Pen G, possess potassium salts and are given by different routes of administration. Pen G is stronger against gram-negative organisms and some anaerobic organisms compared to Pen VK. Pen G is preferred for all infections caused by penicillin-susceptible Streptococcus pneumoniae organisms, gonococcal infections, syphilis, and actinmycosis. Both Pen VK and Pen G are narrow-spectrum penicillins.

Gram+
Adults: loading dose 1 gm, followed by 500 mg every 6 hours for 7–10 days.
Children: < 25 kg: 500 mg, followed by 250 mg every 6 hours.

Aqueous PEN G

Aqueous PEN G is a narrow-spectrum penicillin administered in liquid format. The routes of administration are through intramuscular injection (IM) or intravenous (IV) therapy. Aqueous PEN G is given for infections caused by susceptible microorganisms.

Gram+
Adults: 2 million units every 4–6 hours.
Children: < 50 kg: 100,000–300,000 units/kg/day every 6 hours. Do not exceed adult dose.

Aminopenicillins

Aminopenicillins are broad-spectrum penicillins that will treat gram positive and some gram-negative microorganisms. The two most common aminopenicillins are amoxicillin and ampicillin.

Gram+ and some gram–
Adults: 250–500 mg every 8 hours for 7–10 days.
Children: < 8 years, 20–40 mg/kg/day divided into equal doses every 8 hours.

Erythromycin

Erythromycin inhibits the growth of bacteria and is used as an alternative to penicillin and for acute orofacial infections.

Gram+
Adults: 250–500 mg every 6 hours.
Children: < 25kg: 500 mg, followed by 250 mg every 6 hours.

Clindamycin

Clindamycin binds to the 50S ribosomal subunit and inhibits protein synthesis. Contraindications include liver disorder, renal failure, and blood disorder. Cleocin is a common brand name for clindamycin.

Adults: 150–300 mg every 6 hours for 7–10 days.
Children: < 25kg: 300 mg, followed by 150 mg every 6 hours.

Cephalosporin

Cephalosporin is a broad-spectrum antibiotic that acts against positive and negative bacteria and inhibits cell wall synthesis. Cephalosporin is semi-synthetically produced and used when the patient has a known hypersensitivity to penicillin. Contraindications include allergies/sensitivities and poor renal functions. There are four generations in current use. Keflex is a first-generation cephalosporin known as cephalexin and is the most commonly prescribed cephalosporin.

Adults: 250–500 mg every 6 hours for 7–10 days.
Children: 25–50 mg/kg in divided doses 4 times per day.

TOPICAL ANESTHETICS

Topical anesthetics are used to help decrease patient discomfort for minor procedures or prior to an injection of other anesthesia. They are easier to acquire in the global setting and can be used for immediate but temporary relief of dental pain.

Eugenol (Oil of Clove)

How supplied: gel, liquid vial, or bottle.

Apply directly to the site with a cotton tip applicator, cotton pellet, gauze, or tissue paper. Allow for absorption into the surrounding tissue. Eugenol may be applied to a cotton pellet and placed directly into the tooth. Do not apply a zinc oxide and eugenol mixture directly to an exposed pulp.

Benzocaine 20 Percent
How supplied: gel or topical spray.

Apply directly to the site with a cotton tip applicator, cotton pellet, gauze, or tissue paper. If in an aerosol can, spray with extension tube from 1 to 2 inches away from afflicted site and allow 30 seconds for onset. Check for sensitivity and repeat as needed.

Lidocaine
How supplied: gel or topical spray.

Apply directly to the site with a cotton tip applicator, cotton pellet, gauze, or tissue paper. Effective on the surfaces of the gums and the mucosa.

GENERAL ANESTHESIA

General anesthesia is the administration of hypnotic, sedative, or a combination of medications that will produce a desired effect in the patient in order to perform dental procedures. The use of anesthesia requires an extensive knowledge of the properties of the medication being used, including onset, peak onset, half-life, contraindications, special considerations, complications, and overall duration of the medication.

General anesthesia can be administered several different ways, depending on the medication being used. The most common route is through IV administration. Other administrative routes include oral ingestion and inhalation.

The medical practitioner/operator must monitor the patient for respiratory depression and apnea at all times. Treat signs of respiratory depression and apnea with assisted ventilations using the bag valve mask (BVM).

Midazolam

This general anesthetic is a short-duration sedative hypnotic with amnesia-production qualities.

How supplied: 1 mg/ml in 10 ml vial or 5 mg/ml in 10 ml vial
Administered: IV, IM
Onset: rapid

If overdosed, administer flumazenil.

Ketamine

A general anesthetic with hallucinogenic effects that increase the effects of other sedatives, such as alcoholic beverages, anesthetics, barbiturates, benzodiazepines (Midazolam), and opiates.

How supplied: various concentrations, 50 mg/ml in 10 ml vial, 100 mg/ml in 10 ml vial, 10 mg/ml in 20 ml vial
Administered: IV, IM, PO, rectal, nasal
Onset: rapid

If overdosed, begin aggressive supportive care and treat specific symptoms. Treat respiratory depression with mechanical ventilation (BVM) and supplemental oxygen. If patient experiences seizures, administer short-acting barbiturates or benzodiazepines for sedation. Administer clonidine if hypertension develops. Administer atropine if increased salivation develops.

Propofol

A sedative hypnotic of short duration.

How supplied: 10 mg/ml in 20 ml vial
Administered: IV
Onset: rapid

If overdosed, discontinue use, and treat respiratory depression with mechanical ventilation (BVM) and supplemental oxygen. Treat the patient with atropine if bradycardia and hypotension develops.

Fentanyl

Opioid analgesic of short duration that crosses the blood–brain barrier.

How supplied: 50 mcg/1 ml in 2 ml vial; 25 mcg/hr, 50 mcg/hr, 75 mcg/hr, 100 mcg/hr in transdermal patches; 200 mcg, 400 mcg, 600 mcg, 800 mcg, 1200 mcg, 1600mcg in lozenges
Administered: IV, PO, transdermal, nasal
Onset: rapid

If overdosed, administer Narcan and provide aggressive supportive care. Treat respiratory depression with mechanical ventilation (BVM) and supplemental oxygen, monitor cardiac disturbances, and treat accordingly.

ANESTHETIC INJECTION

Anesthetic injection delivers the appropriate medication to a target location to produce a regional or area-specific block. The anesthetic is deposited in the area nearest the nerve branch and is left to diffuse through the target area to obtain the desired effect of blocking the nerve impulse. By blocking the impulse, the patient should not feel pain during dental procedures.

How supplied: 1.8 ml carpules in blister packs and color-coded.

2 percent lidocaine with epi 1/100,000 (Xylocaine)
Color code: red
Onset: rapid
Duration: 2–4 hours
Max dose with epi: 4.5 mg/kg–7 mg/kg

.5 percent bupivacaine with epi 1/200,000 (Marcaine)
Color code: blue
Onset: slow
Duration: 4–8 hours
Max dose with epi: 2.5 mg/kg–3 mg/kg

3 percent mepivacaine without epi (Carbocaine or Polocaine)
Color code: tan
Onset: rapid
Duration: 20–40 minutes
Max dose: 4–5 mg/kg–7 mg/kg

Procaine (Novocain)
Color code: clear or unmarked
Onset: slow
Duration: 45–90 minutes
Max dose with epi: 8 mg/kg–10 mg/kg

ANESTHETIC INHALATION

The anesthetic inhalation method uses nitrous oxide and oxygen to produce the desired effect in the patient to perform dental procedures. The patient will often state before procedures that he or she prefers a less invasive method to achieve a level of comfort. Anesthetic inhalation provides the necessary level of distraction and comfort for the patient.

For more complicated procedures, anesthetic inhalation will not be sufficient to produce the desired effect in the patient. It can, however, be used as the first line of treatment to gain compliance with the patient before performing the necessary blocks in the oral cavity. Anesthetic inhalation in a remote or austere setting requires more resources than injection, IV, and oral administration. Nonetheless, do not exclude it as a method of treating the patient for pain management and comfort during a dental procedure.

Nitrous oxide (N_2O)

Nitrous oxide readily combines with the patient's hemoglobin and leaves the patient feeling dissociated and euphoric. The administration route is through a specially designed mask that covers the patient's nose and combines with oxygen to flow during procedure. Nitrous oxide is best used for pediatric patients and patients who experience anxiety, low pain tolerance, or mental disorders.

NERVE BLOCKS

Dental nerve blocks are applied to specific areas in the oral cavity to produce a desired effect. The anesthetic is delivered near or close to the target area and deposited in a bubble or linear format. Anesthetic can be deposited at a nerve branch and left to diffuse throughout the target area. After a few minutes, the patient is checked for sensitivity to pain. If the patient does not experience pain when the medical practitioner/operator applies a stimulus to the procedure area, dental procedures can begin.

Several methodologies can be applied to achieve a nerve block. Each method has pros and cons, but the determining factor for choice of application is the proficiency and skill set of the practitioner/operator. It is recommended to learn one method very well instead of learning several methods and applying them with moderate success. The failure of most dental nerve blocks can usually be attributed to operator error rather than the block itself.

Administration techniques for nerve blocks include the following:

- Infiltration—An injection of anesthetic into the tissue immediately surrounding the surgical site.
- Intraseptal—An injection of anesthetic into the papilla of the area to be anesthetized.
- Intraosseous—An injection directly into the tooth's bone structure.
- Intrapulpal—An injection directly into the pulp of the tooth. The tooth becomes desensitized more from pressure of fluid in the chamber than the actual anesthetic.

Inferior Alveolar Nerve Block

The inferior alveolar nerve (IAN) block is the most prevalent technique used by practitioners. It targets the mandibular sulcus. Anatomical landmarks during the procedure are the teeth, pterygomandibular raphe, and retromolar pad.

Even though the IAN block is widely used, it has a reported failure rate as high as 20 percent. Research indicates that the failure to properly anesthetize the patient is largely attributed to improper technique, lack of training, limited mobility of the patient's jaw, and the patient's anatomy making it difficult to locate the mandibular ramus and mandibular foramen.

Many studies have been conducted on the success and failure rates of the IAN block, as well as the Akinosi and Gow-Gates methods. Each methodology has a consistent success ratio when the medical practitioner/operator is properly trained in the technique. The practitioner/operator chooses his or her preferred method based upon his or her level of training and clinical expertise.

Keys to success:

❑ The medical practitioner/operator must approach the target area at the appropriate angle and depth to deposit the anesthetic.
❑ Short needles are recommended for administration of anesthetic because long needles have a tendency to bind.

❏ The targeted nerve must move forward in the mouth for easier accessibility during needle insertion. This is accommodated by opening the patient's mouth as wide as possible.

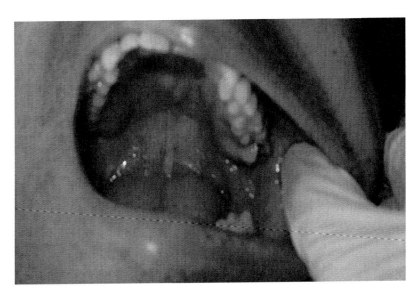

One of the keys to successfully applying an inferior alveolar nerve block is to have the patient open his or her mouth wide.

Methodology

Identify insertion area. Target the mandibular foramen near the medial border of the mandibular ramus and approximately 6 to 10 mm above the biting surfaces of the lower molars.

Place the thumb inside the mouth at the coronoid notch and the index finger outside of the mouth on the posterior border. Pull the buccal soft tissue aside to expose the insertion site. Draw an imaginary line that bisects the thumbnail inside the mouth. This imaginary line will be used to guide the needle into the soft tissue depression.

Place the barrel of the syringe at the opposite end of the mouth on the lower bicuspids and hold parallel to the teeth.

Insert the needle into the V-shaped depression, approximately 25 mm in depth, until bone is contacted. Aspirate for blood. If there is blood present in the hub, reposition the tip of the needle and deposit 0.5 to 1.0 cc of anesthetic. After depositing anesthetic, leave the needle in place and move the barrel to the opposite side of the mouth from where the needle is inserted. Deposit another 0.5 cc of anesthetic as the needle is withdrawn to anesthetize the lingual nerve.

Finish with a long buccal block by depositing approximately 0.5 cc of anesthetic into the buccal mucosa lateral to the third molar.

Allow five minutes for the onset of anesthetic. Check the patient for sensation and then continue with the dental procedure.

Gow-Gates Nerve Block

The Gow-Gates nerve block can be used as a primary technique to anesthetize the mandibular teeth to midline, the floor of the mouth, the tongue to midline, or the tissues and bone of the buccal and lingual. It can also be used as an alternative to the IAN technique if the IAN block fails. The Gow-Gates injection site is set higher than the inferior alveolar nerve. The landmark to help guide needle insertion is the intertragic notch to the corner of the mouth, distal to the second maxillary molar.

Methodology

At the coronoid notch, pull the buccal tissue aside with your hand.

Draw an imaginary line from the intertragic notch to the second maxillary molar. This imaginary line is used to keep the needle parallel as it is advanced to the neck of the condyle. When the needle makes contact with the bone, pull it back approximately 1 mm and aspirate for blood in the hub and barrel of the syringe. If there is no blood, continue with administration of a full carpule of anesthetic. Have the patient remain seated with the mouth open wide to help the anesthetic diffuse into the area of administration.

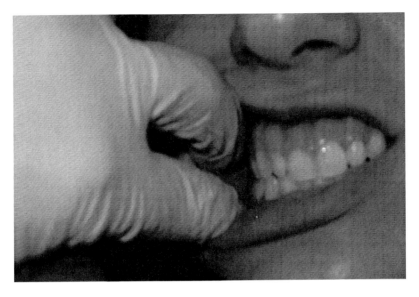

Akinosi nerve block, closed-mouth technique.

Allow the onset of anesthetic to occur within five to seven minutes. Check the patient for sensation and then continue with the dental procedure.

Akinosi Nerve Block

The Akinosi nerve block is a closed-mouth technique. It is best suited for children and patients with a fractured mandible, trismus, or mental disabilities.

Methodology

Insert the needle into the soft tissue over the medial border of the mandibular ramus and next to the maxillary tuberosity. Insert the needle to a depth of 25 mm for an adult. Aspirate for blood in the hub and barrel of the syringe. If there is no blood upon aspiration of the syringe, deposit 1.0 to 1.5 cc of anesthetic.

Allow the onset of anesthetic to occur within five to seven minutes. Check the patient for sensation and then continue with the dental procedure.

Greater Palatine Nerve Block

The greater palatine nerve block is for palatal soft tissue, teeth posterior to the maxillary canine, alveolus, and the hard palate.

Methodology
Use a 27-gauge short needle with the bevel side toward the palate. Palpate the palate for the depression of the foramen, medial from the first and second maxillary molar. Dry the area, wipe with antiseptic, and apply topical anesthetic for at least two to three minutes. Use a cotton tip applicator, elevator, or mirror handle to apply pressure to the site along with needle insertion. Continue applying pressure while slowly advancing the needle and applying a few drops of anesthetic. Continue this process until the palatal bone is reached. The continuous pressure with the cotton tip applicator, elevator, or mirror handle will help desensitize the injection site and add to patient comfort. The palatal injection is very painful to the patient. When contact with the palatal bone is made, aspirate the syringe for blood. If there is no blood present, administer 1/4 to 1/3 carpule of anesthetic.

Nasopalatine Nerve Block
The nasopalatine nerve block is for soft and hard tissue of the maxillary anterior palate, canine to canine. The location of the injection site is the incisive papilla into the incisive foramen. Follow the same methodology as the greater palatine nerve block.

PROCEDURES

The following procedures are the basic fundamentals for emergency dentistry in remote and austere environments. Each dentist and oral surgeon will have different preferred methods, medications, and tools for performing dental procedures. The ones presented in this chapter attempt to reflect the highest standard in dental care in these challenging environments, where resources and trained personnel are scarce.

The ultimate goal in emergency dentistry is to save the tooth for the patient. If the tooth cannot be saved, then every effort is diverted to maintaining structural integrity, managing pain, and preventing the spread of infection into other organ systems.

Each dental procedure is stepped in the manner of saving the tooth and all surrounding tissues. Always stay alert to changes in the patient's condition, and be sure to document accurately.

DENTAL EXAMINATION GUIDELINES

A proper dental examination requires a handful of basic tools:

- dental mirror
- explorer
- gauze sponges
- flashlight/headlamp
- materials for record keeping

The general outline of a dental examination is as follows:

❏ Always document injuries and treatments!
❏ Use a dental mirror and a flashlight/headlamp as needed to inspect areas that are hard to see.
❏ Determine the nature of dental care: emergency, inflammation, infection, or trauma. Begin by obtaining an overall impression of the patient.
❏ Check airway, breathing, and circulation (ABCs).
❏ Visually inspect the head, face, and jaw for deformities, contusions, abrasions, punctures, burns, tenderness, lacerations, and swelling (DCAP BTLS).
❏ Visually inspect and palpate the lips and vestibule for abnormalities and DCAP BTLS.
❏ Visually inspect the entire oral frenula for abnormalities.
❏ Visually inspect and palpate the inside surfaces of the cheeks.
❏ Visually inspect the parotid papilla for any abnormalities.
❏ Document all findings and chart accurately.

INSIDE THE MOUTH

❏ Use a flashlight/headlamp and dental mirror as needed.
❏ Visually inspect and palpate the hard palate and floor of mouth.
❏ Visually inspect the soft palate.
❏ Visually inspect the arches of the tonsil and the oral pharynx.
❏ Examine the ventral and dorsal surfaces of the tongue.
❏ Document all findings and chart accurately.

EXAMINING THE TEETH

❏ Inspect for caries.
❏ Inspect the gingiva for inflammation, redness, swelling, or bleeding. The gingiva should be firm to the touch.

❏ Check teeth for sensitivity to hot, cold, sweets, and pressure.

❏ Inspect for missing, loose, or fragmented teeth.

❏ Monitor the patient's reaction to gentle tapping on a suspected tooth. Compare the suspected tooth to a normal tooth.

❏ Continue the evaluation for evidence of disease or trauma.

❏ Consider dental extraction for airway compromise, irreversible pulpitis, complicated fracture with an exposed pulp, chronic periapical abscess, loose tooth with periodontal abscess, and untreated pericoronitis. It is important to salvage as much dental tissue as possible, to include the tooth, pulp, periodontal ligament, and the involved bone structure.

❏ Caries should be charted and accurately documented with a consistent numbering system for the location of the tooth.

❏ Chart and accurately document missing tooth with a consistent numbering system for the location of the tooth.

REMEMBER! You are providing a *temporary* treatment to help manage pain for the patient. All dental injuries and treatment must be accurately documented. Refer the patient to a dentist when necessary.

PROCEDURES

IMPORTANT: Most procedures require the areas around the tooth and the tooth itself to be as dry as possible. A dry surface provides better bonding of compounds/ionomers and better visibility during treatment procedures. The tongue will be the most difficult to control and may require assistance by retracting it away from the procedure site. Production of saliva is a normal process and is easily controlled with dams or by soaking up the moisture with gauzes/sponges.

Thermal Tests
The sensitivity of a tooth can be tested by applying a hot or cold stimulus. Use a normal tooth for a base of comparison during ther-

mal testing of a suspected tooth. If the suspected tooth does not respond to either a hot or cold stimulus, the pulp is necrotic. Document the findings for response and duration of the pain.

Tools, Cold Test
❑ gauze
❑ cotton tip applicator
❑ cold stimulus (e.g., ice cube, skin refrigerant, ethyl chloride)

Tools, Heat Test
❑ rubber dam
❑ gauze
❑ tongue depressor or handle of a dental instrument
❑ heated liquid (e.g., coffee, tea, water)

Methodology

Cold test: Dry the suspected tooth and the area around it. To aid in keeping saliva from the area, use gauze packs to isolate the tooth. Apply a cold stimulus such as an ice cube or a cotton tip applicator sprayed with ethychloride (skin refrigerant) to the suspected tooth near the base of the gum. If the pulp is inflamed, the patient will continue to experience sensitivity once the cold stimulus has been removed. A healthy tooth will respond to the cold stimulus but will stop once the cold application has been removed.

Heat test: Use a rubber dam to help isolate the tooth to be tested. Apply a warm stimulus such as hot liquid (e.g., water, tea, or coffee) to the suspected tooth. The temperature of the liquid should not exceed 140°F to prevent burning the patient. If the patient has a continued painful response after the heat stimulus has been removed, pulpitis can be suspected. If the pain is severe and is relieved by a cold application, the pulp is inflamed and the patient needs a root canal.

PROCEDURES

Draining Tooth Abscess

Pus can accumulate along the borders of the gum line and the root of a tooth due to infection. The accumulation will exert pressure on the tooth and may ultimately displace it from the normal occlusal position. The patient will describe the sensation of the affected tooth feeling "high" because it will be the first to strike before the rest of the teeth come into contact.

If the abscess is left untreated, the patient will experience continuing symptoms of fever, malaise, anorexia, and pain. If the abscess remains untreated, it will require antibiotics to treat the associated infection. The tooth should be extracted as a last resort.

Tools
- ❏ scalpel
- ❏ gauze
- ❏ drainage material (gauze, surgical tubing, t-shaped drain)
- ❏ hemostat
- ❏ suture material (absorbable suture preferred)

Methodology

Administer a local anesthetic. In a cold or arctic environment, application of snow or ice to the fluctuant area may be enough to manage the pain. Once the area has been desensitized, make an incision down to the bone. Perform a blunt dissection of the incision with a hemostat to help increase drainage. Suture a drain into the incision using a T-shape drainage, surgical tubing, gauze, or a finger cut from a surgical glove. Allow the site to drain for two to three days.

If the tooth is decayed, use a spoon-shaped instrument to remove the decay. Make an opening to the pulp chamber. Once the opening is complete, apply pressure to the gingiva with the fingers. Apply pressure closest to the root of the affected tooth to force the pus through the opening that was created. Drain as much pus from the area as the technique will permit. Advise the patient to rinse his or her mouth with a warm saline solution every 2 hours. For pain management, administer 800 mg ibuprofen as needed.

Intraoral Splinting

Intraoral splinting is needed after any procedure that requires the affected tooth to be stabilized. The stabilization is accomplished by adjoining the affected tooth to a nearby healthy tooth that is on the same alveolar ridge. If the medical practitioner/operator does not stabilize the affected tooth appropriately, the patient will continue to experience pain, the healing process will be extended, and the tooth may be lost. The purpose of dental work is to save as much viable tissue as possible, in this case, the tooth.

Tools

There are numerous methodologies to help stabilize an affected tooth to a healthy, adjoining tooth. Refer to the individual methodologies below for the required tools for each procedure.

Methodology

Wire: Splint the affected tooth to the two adjacent teeth with wire suture material or a heavy-gauge wire. A paper clip with blunted ends or a safety pin with the ends removed and blunted can be used to splint the affected tooth. Blunting the ends must be done to ensure that the patient's tongue, gingiva, or soft tissue is not lacerated. Glue the wire, safety pin, or paper clip to the affected tooth and the two adjacent teeth for stability and support.

Cotton fibers: Add cotton fibers or strands of fiber from cotton gauze to a zinc oxide and eugenol mix to strengthen the splint. Form the mixture to the affected tooth and mold it to the two adjacent teeth for stability and support. Fill the spaces and voids between the teeth with the mixture.

Suture: Use sutures to hold the affected tooth in place. Place sutures around the tooth and through the gum for stability and support. Absorbable sutures are highly recommended for simplicity and streamlining the patient load in forward areas, remote clinics, and austere environments.

SAM splints: Use a SAM splint for splinting the affected tooth to the two adjacent teeth. Cut the splint into small, thin strips and apply to the affected tooth with a nontoxic glue or stomadhesive. Ensure there are no sharp edges to the SAM splint to avoid laceration of the tongue, gingiva, or soft tissue.

Candle wax: Soften candle wax and mold into place to act as a splint. This method requires consistent monitoring to ensure that the splint holds. This method is the least reliable but will serve as a temporary splint in the absence of a more durable splinting procedure. Heat the candle wax until it becomes pliable and then mold it over the affected tooth and to the two adjacent teeth for stability and support. Fill in the spaces and voids to ensure the splint remains in place for a longer duration.

Transporting a Tooth

The goal of tooth transportation is to preserve as much viable tissue as possible for reimplantation into the socket. A completely avulsed tooth can be reimplanted into the socket if done within an hour time frame. To increase the chance of success for reimplantation, minimize handling of the tooth, and do not attempt to scale or scrape off debris from the tooth. This reduces the risk of damaging the periodontal ligament and possibly removing it from the avulsed tooth. When handling the tooth, hold it by the crown and gently rinse it with 0.9 percent normal saline.

If immediate reimplantation cannot be achieved in the field, the tooth should be transported in a clean liquid medium. It is very important that the tooth does *not* dry out. Hank's balanced salt solution, saline, contact lens solution, and ordinary white milk are excellent transport mediums. These liquids can be placed in a plastic bag, 35 mm film canister, or 20 ml multidose saline vial. Do not transport the tooth in acidic liquids such as bleach, fruit juices, or disinfectants.

If commercially available preservation mediums are not available,

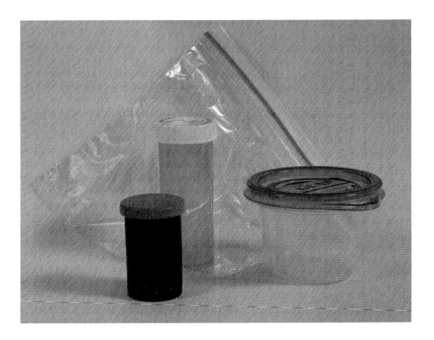

Sample plastic containers in which to transport an avulsed tooth for reimplantation.

alternate methodologies can be used to transport the tooth. Cover the tooth in the transport container with the patient's saliva, or place the tooth underneath the tongue or in the buccal sulcus and transport. If using the latter methodology, give the patient specific instructions not to swallow, and watch the patient for aspiration of the tooth.

Scaling and Cleaning

Brushing and flossing are not always enough to remove the plaque buildup from around the tooth. An extensive cleaning process may be required to remove the tartar from around the base of the tooth and the gum pockets.

The scaling process is time consuming and may require two sessions instead of one. If the patient must return for a second session, scale half of the mouth on one day and the other half when the patient is able to return on another day. Have the patient return when he or she is able to tolerate the second session. The second session should be done as soon as possible.

Keep the scaling tools sterile to prevent transmission of blood-borne pathogens such as hepatitis from one patient to another. Never allow the scaler to become dull. A sharp tool reduces the number of strokes needed to scale around the tooth, and the sharp edges will allow the scaler to cut through the tarter buildup and get closer to the actual surface of the tooth for better cleaning.

Tools
- ❏ C-1 scaler
- ❏ G-11/12 curette
- ❏ dental mirror
- ❏ probe (explorer)
- ❏ tweezers
- ❏ cotton gauze
- ❏ sharpening stone
- ❏ light

Methodology
Advise the patient on the procedure and what is to be expected. The patient should be informed that there will be bleeding and the possibility of a little pain and discomfort. Advise the patient that the procedure will be conducted at his or her pace.

Have the patient lie back on a chair or improvised bench. It is important that the technician and the patient are comfortable for the duration of the procedure.

Use the probe to feel just below the gum line for tartar buildup. Press cotton gauze between the teeth and at the base of the gum line to expose more tartar buildup. The gauze will also serve as a means to absorb excessive saliva during the procedure.

Place the sharp edge of the scaler into the gum pocket and underneath the tartar. Use the sharp edge to remove tartar and debris from the tooth. Deep gum pockets are signs of infections that will remain if all the tartar and debris are not removed. In one smooth motion, pull the scaler up from the root toward the crown of the tooth. Maintain close contact with the surface of the tooth at all times. Use the fewest number of strokes needed to scale the tooth. Unnecessary strokes should be limited to avoid impacting tartar against the surface of the tooth. The impacted tartar will make it harder to completely clean the tooth.

Use the probe to check the surface of the tooth for smoothness. When all the surfaces of the tooth are smooth from the scaling procedure, move onto the next tooth. Continue the process until completely finished. If the patient is unable to continue, do half of the mouth and have the patient return when he or she is able to.

Control any bleeding by applying direct pressure with gauze.

When the session is completed, advise the patient on proper oral hygiene. Demonstrate proper brushing and flossing techniques. The patient must be dedicated to maintaining proper oral hygiene, or the

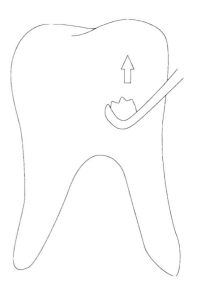

Proper direction for scaling, from the root to the crown.

scaling session will have been in vain. The tartar will continue to build up and infection will reoccur.

Have the patient continue with warm saltwater rinses.

Advise the patient on how to strengthen the gums with a proper diet of fruits and vegetables.

Remember: Do not rush the procedure!

Atraumatic Restorative Treatment (ART)

Atraumatic restorative treatment (ART) has several advantages for the medical practitioner operating in remote, disaster, or austere settings. The technique is used primarily where electricity is not available and the possibility of causing pain to the patient is very low. Missionary work, disaster relief, forward clinics, Special Forces "hearts and minds" campaigns, humanitarian aid projects, and austere environments benefit from this technique due to its high success rate and the low training time needed for the medical practitioner/operator to achieve consistent performance and proficiency.

Other advantages include the simplicity of the technique and the few tools required. Each practitioner/operator can customize their kit for deployment and mission-specific needs. Fewer tools means tremendous weight savings for the practitioner/operator traveling by foot to remote regions. ART rarely requires anesthetic application for pain, although it sometimes is needed due to lack of training on the part of the practitioner/operator or insistence of the patient. Regardless, this technique is largely painless and is used on children with a great deal of success.

From the standpoint of aesthetic appeal, the sealant used in ART bonds well with the tooth and is generally the same color as the tooth. Each filling is cost effective per patient being treated because it seals the affected tooth, provides fluoride that will kill the remaining decay, and protects against secondary decay.

Tools
❏ Fuji IX ionomer
❏ dental spatula, #24

- ❏ spoon evacuator, #36/37
- ❏ dental hatchet
- ❏ dental explorer
- ❏ dental mirror
- ❏ dental mixing pad
- ❏ Woodson pluggers, #2 or #3
- ❏ Tofflemire matrix bands, .0010 dead soft
- ❏ Tofflemire matrix band holders
- ❏ small can of compressed air if available, or a bulb syringe
- ❏ light source

NOTE: For this procedure, a portable handheld electric dental drill (30-40, #245 burs) can be used. It will be discussed as an option below.

Methodology

Tooth selection: Select the proper tooth. The tooth identified should *not* be sensitive to pain or have swelling around the surrounding tissues. The tooth may be sensitive to hot or cold application but should not elicit an immediate painful response from the patient.

Option: ART is a technique that should not cause pain, but keep anesthetic delivery as a viable option for patient comfort when needed. Medical practitioners/operators have noted incidents where anesthetic delivery was needed or suggested.

Tooth preparation: Remove plaque from the surface of the tooth with moist cotton pellets or moist cotton gauze. When the plaque has been removed, dry the tooth and surrounding area thoroughly. The treatment area should be kept as dry as possible for the best adhesion of the restoration. Compressed air can be used to help dry the area and clear away debris from the procedure site.

Use a dental hatchet to remove the enamel and decayed dentin from the tooth. Sometimes it will be necessary to create a larger opening for the restoration.

Option: Use a portable handheld dental drill to remove the

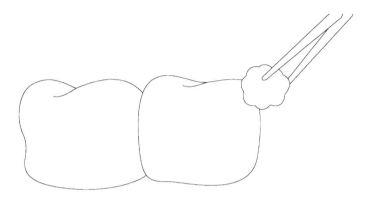

Removing plaque from the procedure site with moist cotton.

enamel and decayed dentin. Work in a circular motion, and do not exceed the cutting surface of the bur.

Remove carious lesion: Use the spoon evacuator to remove as much of the carious lesion as possible. Irrigate the cavity with warm water or use compressed air to remove debris. Isolate the tooth with gauze packs and dry it with cotton pellets. Remember to keep the area dry for better bonding.

Apply the Fuji IX: Use a Woodson instrument or a moist cotton tip applicator to tamp the mixture into the tooth with quick repeated jabs. Air bubbles may form at any time during the procedure but can be reduced significantly with the repeated jabbing/tamping process. Once the mixture has been tamped into place, excess must be removed. Use a wet, gloved hand or a moist cotton pellet to remove the excess mixture by rubbing the material away from the tooth. Alternatively, a medium/large excavator can be used to scrape the excess mixture away from the tooth.

There are other commercially available alternatives for the filling, but Fuji IX is recommended due to its widespread availability on the global market.

If Fuji IX is unavailable, alternative temporary fillings include the following:

1. Mix zinc oxide powder and 2 to 3 drops of eugenol for approximately 1 minute to form a putty. Apply the putty to the restoration by using the same jabbing/tamping method with a cotton tip applicator or Woodson instrument to reduce air bubbles and increase adhesion. Allow the putty to harden for 5 to 10 minutes.
2. Soak a cotton pellet with eugenol and place into the cavity.
3. Soften candle wax and set into cavity to help protect the pulp.

Set and harden: Allow time for the filling to set and harden. It is vital for the tooth and procedure area to remain dry during this time frame.

Check the bite: After 1 to 2 minutes, check the patient's bite. Have the patient bite down several times to ensure that the restoration is not too high and the tooth seats properly in the normal occlusal plane for chewing.

Advise patient: The patient should not eat or chew on the affected side for at least an hour.

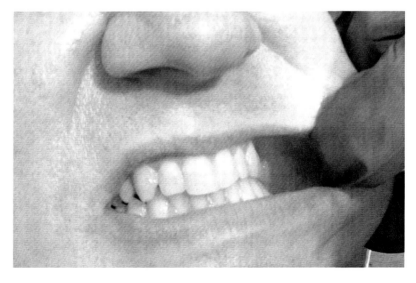

Have the patient bite down to check the positioning of the restoration.

Extracting a Tooth

When extracting a tooth, the general principle is to use an elevator of choice, such as a 12B, to loosen the tooth and a combination of forceps to complete the extraction. Inspect the socket for any fragments that may have broken off from the root, manage bleeding, and advise and educate the patient.

Tools

❏ anesthesia equipment
❏ surgical forceps:
    ✓ 150 for maxillary anterior and bicuspids
    ✓ 151 for mandibular anterior and bicuspids
    ✓ 17 for mandibular molars
    ✓ 53L for maxillary left molars
    ✓ 53R for maxillary right molars
❏ elevators

Methodology

Assess the patient and obtain his or her medical history and allergies. Explain what to expect and the procedure involved. Gather and assemble equipment, and identify the tooth or teeth to be extracted.

After administering the appropriate anesthetic, use an elevator to break the attachment of gingival tissue to the tooth. Force the tips of the forceps into the gingival margin and apply pressure toward the root of the tooth. This will help to get the tips of the forceps farther down the root.

Start by using a slow, rocking motion to loosen the tooth; then increase the tempo of the rocking action. A facial-lingual (side to side) direction should be used.

Multi-root teeth should be moved in a facial-lingual direction. Do not apply rotational movement to a tooth with more than one root. Single-root teeth, however, can be loosened with both a rocking and rotational motion.

Once the tooth is loose, apply gentle traction to remove it in the direction of least resistance.

Inspect the tooth for completeness. Make sure that the root did not become fractured and fragmented. Portions of the tooth may be imbedded in the socket. Inspect the socket for any fragments.

Manage bleeding by compressing the sides of the empty socket. Apply folded, 2 x 2 gauze to the wound and have the patient maintain bite pressure for 30 minutes or longer. There are also hemostatic agents available to help control the bleeding.

Advise the patient not to rinse the mouth for the next 12 hours.

Explain to the patient *not* to disturb the clot. Advise the patient to avoid eating foods that are hard, hot, or spicy for a few days.

Schedule follow-up care.

Following these guidelines will help the patient to minimize post-extraction complications.

TRAUMA

Dental trauma can occur inside and outside and at different levels of the oral cavity. Most dental traumas are associated with impact sports or previous medical history of associated trauma. When examining a patient with dental trauma, first check that the airway is clear of obstructions. Once the ABCs have been addressed, examination and treatment of the trauma may proceed.

DISLOCATION OF THE TEMPOROMANDIBULAR JOINT

Temporomandibular joint (TMJ) dislocation is caused by the movement of the mandibular condyle to the anterior position of the articular eminence. The dislocation remains locked in this position until reduction and stabilization occurs. TMJ dislocation may occur from eating, yawning, or a dental procedure. Patients with previous history of trauma to the jaw can be suspected of a condyle fracture. The patient may present with a unilateral or bilateral dislocation of the TMJ. Muscle spasms may also prevent the patient from closing his or her mouth.

Treatment
Start reduction and stabilization of the dislocation as soon as possible.

Methodology

Always allow the process to naturally occur if the patient is able to self-reduce. Applying heat packs or moist heat to both sides of the jaw may help the patient to self-reduce the dislocation.

If the patient is unable to self reduce, you will have to perform manual reduction. Muscle spasms may be severe and will complicate the reduction. The patient will require sedation prior to manual reduction. Administer Diazepam or Midazolam (Versed). Have the patient sit down or lie down. If the patient is sitting down on a chair, stand behind the patient and stabilize his or her head against the chair, wall, or your torso. If the patient is lying down, place yourself on the ground with the head lying in your lap for stabilization.

Wrap your thumbs with gauze or small strips of cloth to protect them from being bitten accidentally. Grab the mandible with the fingers and place the wrapped thumbs inside the patient's mouth behind the last molars. With firm, steady pressure, push down and back with the thumbs while maintaining upward pressure at the chin. The condyle will pass over the crest of the TMJ and slide back into position with a "clunk" sound. It is very important to maintain pressure on the chin to hold the teeth and jaw in position.

CAUTION: The patient can still easily dislocate the TMJ due to the natural desire to open the mouth. Secure the jaw closed once dislocation has been reduced. Wrap a bandage or cling around the patient's chin and top of the head and secure in place.

Refer to definitive care with an oral surgeon if continued dislocation occurs or you are unable to reduce dislocation. Advise the patient to avoid talking, chewing, and yawning for a few hours to help prevent the jaw from dislocating again.

LACERATIONS

All lacerations should be inspected for tooth fragments, debris, and other foreign bodies. Small lacerations of the gingiva and buccal mucosa will heal quickly and without too much dental intervention.

Cold compresses, gauze, hemostatic agents, direct pressure, and ice are simple methods to help control bleeding.

Lacerations larger than 1 to 2 cm will require sutures to close the wound. Approximate the edges of the lacerations using 4-0 or 5-0 absorbable sutures. The suture knots should be buried beneath the surface. If nonabsorbable sutures are used to close the wound, they must be inspected and removed after the wound has healed.

When selecting sutures for wounds of the gingiva or the buccal mucosa, use suture material that causes the least amount of tissue damage and irritation.

CRACKED ENAMEL (CRAZE)

Small lines or cracks that penetrate the enamel or both the enamel and dentin is known as crazing. The craze can damage the structure of hard tissue but will *not* result in tissue loss. The tooth will be very sensitive to hot and cold applications.

Treatment
Cover the crack with a dental varnish or nail polish. Ensure that any nail polish application is nontoxic to the patient.

CONCUSSION/CONTUSION

This is when the tooth is permanently bruised. Blood in the dentin will give the tooth a brownish color, and percussion and pressure will cause the tooth to be tender. The tooth will not be mobile in the socket. No manipulation of the tooth is required and should be avoided.

Treatment
Apply ice pack and administer nonsteroidal anti-inflammatory drugs (NSAIDs).

TOOTH FRACTURES

There are several different ways to classify a tooth fracture. Within the emergency medicine community, the Ellis classification system is the most commonly used. Another method is through simple description of the tooth fracture. Many medical practitioners/operators are able to understand and pass along information based upon this method. Simple description does not require extensive training and is easily understood by different levels of medical practitioners/operators and the patient.

The Ellis classification system identifies three types of dental fractures.

- Ellis Class I—Uncomplicated fractures of the crown that involve only the enamel.
- Ellis Class II—Uncomplicated fractures of the crown that involve the enamel and the dentin but not the pulp.
- Ellis Class III—Complicated fractures of the crown that involve the enamel, dentin, and pulp. An Ellis Class III is a true dental emergency.

Fractures will occur at different levels of the tooth. All fractures can affect the bone structure and the socket. Any trauma can lead to the loss of the tooth or extensive damage to the bone structure. Monitor the patient for airway compromise.

Simple Crown Fractures–Ellis Class I

Simple crown fractures–Ellis Class I are uncomplicated fractures of the crown that involve the enamel only. The tooth may be chipped or missing large sections of enamel.

The patient will complain of rough or sharp edges around the tooth. Pain is not commonly associated with simple fractures, but sensitivity to heat and cold applications may be noted. The front incisors are commonly involved in simple crown fractures.

Treatment

Use a small flat file, emery board, or rotary disk sander to smooth the rough edges of the tooth. Inspect the areas of the lips, tongue, and gingiva for any tooth fragments that may be embedded. Apply cavity varnish over the broken tooth. Advise the patient to follow up with a dentist for restoration of the tooth.

Simple Crown Fractures–Ellis Class II Uncomplicated

The Ellis Class II is similar to Class I but extends into the dentin. The patient will complain of pain and sensitivity to heat, cold, or air. Examination of the tooth will reveal a yellowish tint of the dentin versus the white color of the enamel. The tooth will have rough and sharp edges without exposure of the pulp. Fractures that are close to the pulp should be monitored closely. The bacteria of the oral cavity can pass through the pores of the dentin and cause inflammation and infection of the pulp. Treat children with this condition more aggressively than adults because of the possibility of bacteria spreading and causing an infection.

Treatment

Rinse the tooth with a warm saline solution. Isolate the area with cotton rolls or gauze. Dry the area and the affected tooth very carefully with gauze or cotton pellets. Apply several coats of zinc oxide and eugenol paste over the tooth. Cotton fibers can be added to the mixture for additional strength. A calcium hydroxide paste or glass ionomer can also be used. It is recommended to place a foil covering over the tooth to prevent the dressing from becoming dislodged or if there is an extended time frame before the patient can be seen by definitive dental care. Cut, trim, and contour the foil covering to fit. Ensure that the gingiva will not be lacerated by the foil. Splint the tooth to the adjacent teeth for additional strength and support.

Advise the patient to eat a soft diet. The patient should avoid hard food and sticky candy such as gum or taffy. The patient should also avoid hot or cold fluids and chewing on the fractured tooth to reduce the chances of dislodging the dressing.

Complicated Crown/Root Fractures–Ellis Class III

Complicated crown/root fractures are true emergencies that involve the enamel, dentin, and pulp. The fractured tooth should be wiped with gauze to allow visual inspection for the pink coloration of the pulp. The patient will complain of severe to excruciating pain.

Treatment

Control bleeding. Anesthetize the tooth and begin irrigating the area with a warm saline solution. Remove all loose fragments of tooth from the area, to include the buccal tissue, gingiva, tongue, and lips. Isolate the tooth with cotton rolls or gauze. Dry the tooth thoroughly with cotton pellets. Consider removing up to 2 mm of necrotic pulp if the exposure is greater than 24 hours. Apply Dycal, intermediate restorative material (IRM), glass ionomer, or candle wax sealant to cover the pulp and allow time for the dressing to harden. Inspect the area for tooth impact that may irritate the surrounding tissue or trap food and debris. Cover with stomadhesive and advise the patient to adhere to a liquid diet. The patient must be seen by a dentist as soon as possible. Special consideration should be given to extracting the tooth.

Do not apply zinc oxide and eugenol to an exposed pulp. The application will kill the pulp.

ROOT FRACTURES

Root fractures occur below the gum line and may involve more than one root and the bone structure. It may take several months for the bone to heal. Exposed pulp should be sealed as part of the treatment process. Root fractures are sometimes difficult to distinguish from a luxation and may require an X-ray. The crown may be partially or fully broken. If the crown is totally broken, do not attempt to extract the root.

Treatment

Reposition the tooth. Remove all fragments, stabilize the tooth, and splint with wires and stomadhesive.

Do not apply zinc oxide and eugenol to an exposed pulp. The application will kill the pulp.

LUXATIONS AND SUBLUXATIONS

Luxations are teeth that are displaced from their original position and will move with the bone. The condition may result from trauma or injury to the periodontal ligament and gingiva. The type of luxation is indicated by movement of the tooth in a specific direction. A lateral luxation will result in movement of the tooth facially, mesially, lingually, or distally. The tooth remains intact, but the root is displaced from the normal position and breaks the bone.

Subluxations are teeth that move within the socket or are loose but are not displaced.

Treatment

Luxations require manual movement of the tooth back into the normal occlusal position. Administer a local anesthetic for pain management. A knot is located at the area of displacement. Place one finger at the tip of the tooth and another finger near the knot. Pull the tooth at the tip and push at the root to push the tooth back into place. Splint the tooth to the adjacent teeth with wire, a paper clip with blunted ends, heavy fishing line, IRM/cotton fiber, glass ionomer, or stomadhesive. This will help to hold the tooth and bone in place. Advise the patient to avoid chewing on the affected side.

Subluxations will not require manual manipulation but should be splinted to the adjacent teeth.

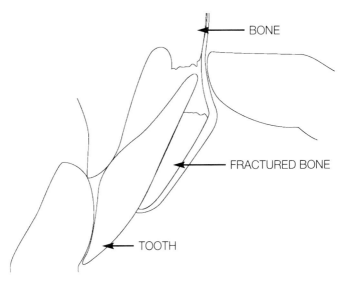

BONE

FRACTURED BONE

TOOTH

An example of a luxation. Manual manipulation in a cantilever motion is required to move the tooth back into the normal occlusal plane.

INTRUSION

An intrusion occurs when a tooth has been impacted deeper into the socket. The intrusion can result in a crushing injury of the periodontal ligament and the vascular supply of the pulp. The intrusion may fracture the tooth and the alveolar ridge.

Treatment
The patient must see a dentist. Pain management may require extraction of the tooth. Apply dental first aid to provide patient comfort.

EXTRUSION

An extrusion occurs when a tooth has been pulled out from the socket and displays movement. The medical practitioner/operator must rule out an avulsion or fracture. Gently pull on the tooth to identify if the tooth is an extrusion.

Treatment
Push the tooth back into the socket. Apply stomadhesive and splint to adjacent teeth for added support. Have the patient bite down to ensure that the tooth is seated properly in the socket.

AVULSED TOOTH

An avulsed tooth is completely removed from the socket and is a true dental emergency. A visual inspection will reveal an empty socket where the tooth would be. The first question the medical practitioner/operator should ask is, "Where is the tooth?" The patient may have the tooth in hand upon presentation to the medical practitioner/operator. If the tooth is not present, ask the patient if he or she had been coughing, had consumed alcoholic beverages, and about the activities leading to the avulsion. The tooth may be embedded in the oral mucosa, fractured, swallowed, or aspirated. Inspect the alveolar ridge and socket for deformities and fractures. If the alveolar ridge is fractured or the socket has sustained extensive injuries and damage, do not attempt to reimplant the tooth. Some avulsions may require X-rays to locate the missing tooth. For children with primary tooth avulsion, the tooth should not be reimplanted.

The goal is to reimplant an avulsed tooth in the shortest possible time frame with a viable, healthy periodontal ligament. Success of reimplantation is greater if done within an hour of the avulsion. The avulsed tooth may be immersed in Doxycycline prior to reimplantation. The immersion may help prevent external root resorption. Minimize handling of the tooth, and hold the tooth only by the crown.

Treatment

ABC's first!

Control bleeding with any of the following methodology:

❏ Direct pressure with gauze.

❏ Moist tea bag application into the socket.

❏ Hemostatic agents such as ActCel or Celox.

Gently irrigate debris from the tooth with a 0.9 percent saline solution. *Do not* attempt to scale or scrape the tooth. This will reduce the chance of removing the periodontal ligament from the tooth.

Gently irrigate the socket to remove blood clots and trapped debris. Anesthetize the area as needed for patient comfort and pain management. After the anesthesia has taken effect, place the tooth into the socket with slow, steady pressure.

Splint the tooth by suturing in place through the gum, splinting with wires to the adjacent teeth, or covering with stomadhesive or an IRM/cotton fiber mix. Refer the patient to a dentist.

To manage mild pain for an avulsed tooth, administer acetaminophen or ibuprofen. For severe pain, administer acetaminophen with codeine. Do not use aspirin to manage pain. Administer an antibiotic regimen as appropriate for the area of operation.

INFLAMMATION

Dental inflammation is the body's response to a foreign body. The inflammation can be acute or chronic. It is often characterized by swelling, redness, and pain at the site. Early treatment of dental inflammation may prevent the inflammation from becoming an infection. The common causes of dental inflammation are trauma, allergies, bacteria, virus, or chemical exposure.

ALVEOLAR OSTEITIS

Alveolar osteitis (dry socket) occurs when the alveolar bone becomes inflamed post extraction of a tooth. The inflammation occurs because a clot fails to form, dissolves, or becomes dislodged. Contributing factors include smoking, hormone therapy, age (older than 25 years), periodontal disease, traumatic extractions, or impacted third molars (wisdom tooth).

The patient will complain of severe and constant pain that radiates from the ear to the lower jaw. The pain begins two to four days after a tooth extraction. Further presentation will include an exposed alveolar bone, foul mouth odor, and debris and food particles seen in the socket without the formed clot.

Treatment
Manage the patient's pain with NSAIDs. If the pain is not re-

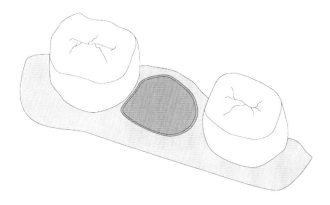

Alveolar osteitis (dry socket) is is an empty space, postextraction of a tooth that has become inflammed.

lieved, consider using a dental block. Once the pain is managed, re-move accumulated debris and food particles with a warm saline rinse. Use gentle suction with a bulb syringe or mechanical suction if available.

Apply two to three drops of eugenol (oil of cloves) to an approx-imate 2-inch strip of iodoform gauze. Pack the impregnated gauze loosely into the socket. Avoid applying excessive pressure on the socket. Repack the socket every 24 hours for a period of five to seven days.

Alternate packing options include a Gelfoam/eugenol slurry or Gelfoam with dry socket paste. The Gelfoam and dry socket paste will stay in place longer than gauze due to the thickness of the slurry.

CARIES

Dental caries (cavities) is a common bacterial disease of the teeth. The disease begins to destroy the enamel and dentin of the affected tooth due to the buildup of plaque. Prolonged exposure to the acidic by-products of plaque will continue to break down the tooth's enamel. This process can take months to years before a cavity begins to form. The patient's diet and oral hygiene have a large impact on the progression of the disease. Most dental caries can be reversed if recognized and treated in the early stages.

The caries will initially appear whitish in color, with gray undertones on the enamel of the tooth. As the disease continues, the enamel and dentin will change color. The tooth will appear brown and the dentin will be spongy, soft, and yellowish in color. Dark stains on the tooth are not always indications of caries; some dark stains are attributed to the patient's diet.

Caries are the most common cause of dental pain. The patient will complain of sensitivity to cold, sweets, salts, and pressure when biting/chewing, as well as intermittent to continuous pain.

Treatment

Locate the offending tooth. Use a normal tooth for a comparison of responses when conducting tests. The carious tooth will elicit a painful response from the patient when tapped with an instrument. Check tooth vitality by touching the dentin or applying a cold stimulus. Both methods should elicit a painful response and subside once the stimulus has been removed. This will indicate a vital tooth. If a painful response is noted during application of a heat stimulus, the pulp may be necrotic or dead.

Remove the caries with a spoon excavator and flush the cavity with warm water. Dry the treatment area with cotton pellets and control the saliva around the area. Maintain a dry treatment area for better adhesion of the restoration. Administer local anesthetic as needed for patient pain and discomfort. Fill the cavity with a temporary zinc oxide and eugenol filling or IRM. Allow the filling to dry and harden. Have the patient bite down repeatedly to check for normal occlusion. Remove excess material from around the tooth.

Never apply a zinc oxide and eugenol mix directly to a vital pulp. This mixture will kill the pulp.

PULPITIS

Reversible pulpitis is an inflammation caused by caries that intrudes upon the dental pulp. The patient will complain of tension, pressure, and hot and cold sensitivity. The patient may be unable to identify the location of the exact tooth. If the caries progresses without intervention, the inflammation will become severe and change to irreversible pulpitis. The irreversible pulpitis will require a root canal or extraction of the offending tooth.

Treatment
Remove the caries with a spoon excavator and flush the cavity with warm water. Dry the treatment area with cotton pellets and control the saliva around the area. Maintain a dry treatment area for better adhesion of the restoration. Administer local anesthetic as needed for patient pain and discomfort. Fill the cavity with a temporary zinc oxide and eugenol filling or IRM. Allow the filling to dry and harden. Have the patient bite down repeatedly to check for normal occlusion. Remove excess material from around the tooth. Candle wax can be softened and placed over the tooth to protect the nerve until definitive care can be obtained.

Do not apply a zinc oxide and eugenol mix to a vital pulp. This mixture will kill the pulp.

GINGIVITIS

The gingiva (gum) is the soft tissue surrounding the tooth. It feels firm to the touch and fits close to the tooth. When the gingiva becomes inflamed, the gums will become swollen and red in appearance. Bleeding may be present around the gum line.

Treatment

Prevention is the first step. Stress proper oral hygiene by teaching brushing and flossing techniques. The medical practitioner/operator may elect to scale the teeth. Advise the patient to frequently rinse his or her mouth with a warm saline solution.

PERICORONITIS

Pericoronitis is an inflammation of the gingival flap over a partially erupted tooth such as the third molar (wisdom tooth). Impact from an opposing tooth can cause the tissue to become inflamed. Food and debris may also be trapped in the gingival flap.

The patient will complain of pain that involves the ears, throat, and mouth, as well as fever, fatigue, muscle spasms of the jaw, and trismus. The gums will be swollen, tender, and red, with localized suppurative over the affected tooth.

Treatment

Use a cotton tip applicator dipped in 3 percent peroxide to clean debris and food particles from underneath the tissue flap. Pus may be present and should be removed from the site by irrigation or gentle suction. Use a syringe and catheter with a warm saline solution to irrigate the area and underneath the tissue. Advise the patient to continue with hot saline solution rinses every two hours until the inflammation begins to clear. Educate the patient on proper oral hygiene and diet. Severe pericoronitis with fever, cervical nodes involvement, and trismus is treated with an antibiotic regimen of penicillin 500 mg or Erythromycin 500 mg every six hours. Consider extraction of the opposing molar if needed.

INFECTION

Dental infection is the progression of a dental injury that is spreading to other parts of the body, as well as the tooth, bone, and soft tissue. The infection may be due to trauma, virus, bacteria, fungus, allergies, or chemical exposure. The bacteria or foreign body may cascade into the patient's systemic or respiratory system. The patient will typically present with fever, malaise, and pain and have associated pus at or around the infection site.

ORAL HERPES

Oral herpes (cold sores; fever blisters) is highly contagious, and preventive measures should be taken to prevent the spread of the virus to other people. Very small ulcers will appear in clusters on the oral mucosa, palate, or near the teeth. The ulcers will initially appear as bright red and will have a flat to slightly raised border. In later stages, the ulcers will have a white plaque covering. The patient will complain of pain, itching, and burning.

Contributing factors include a suppressed immune system, stress, upper respiratory infections, improper diet, vitamin deficiencies, allergies, and trauma to the oral mucosa. In children, oral herpes will cause severe dehydration and anorexia because the child will not want to aggravate the site due to pain.

Treatment

Prevent the spread of infection to other people. Advise the patient to wash hands and avoid touching areas such as the eyes or nose. The patient should not engage in sexual activities, kissing, or touching with partners, family members, and other people. Medication consists of acyclovir 5 percent applied topically to ulcers every 3 hours; benzocaine 20 percent or viscous lidocaine 1 or 2 percent topical anesthetic applied to reduce discomfort; and Tylenol PO for pain and low-grade fever. Infection usually lasts for two weeks.

APHTHOUS ULCERS

Aphthous ulcers (canker sores) are lesions that appear as open sores inside the mouth and around the upper throat. The patient will complain of burning, itching, or stinging with extreme pain. The ulcers will be round in shape, with a white to yellowish color surrounded by an inflamed red border. Three types of ulcerations are noted: minor ulcerations, major ulcerations, and herpetiform ulcerations. Contributing factors include physical trauma, stress, history of ulcerations, immune system deficiencies, vitamin deficiencies, and food allergies.

Minor ulcerations are 2 to 3 mm to several centimeters in diameter. The ulcers are painful and can cause swelling of the affected lip. Typical duration for minor ulcerations is 10 to 14 days.

Major ulcerations have the same presentation as minor ulcers but are larger in diameter. The ulcers have a longer healing time that could last several weeks and will leave a scar.

Herpetiform ulcerations have lesions that are 1 to 2 mm and appear in clusters. The patient will present with a history of recurring lesions. The lesions will heal in 7 to 10 days without scarring.

Treatment

Apply topical steroid fluocinonide 0.5 percent mixed with Orabase to each ulcer six to eight times per day. Alternative medica-

INFECTION

tions include Kenalog in Orabase, Lidex Gel, or Decadron rinses. Advise the patient on proper diet, rest, and fluid intake.

PERIODONTAL ABSCESS

A periodontal abscess is an infection near the root of a tooth that involves the alveolar bone, periodontal ligament, and gingiva. The abscess will appear closest to the side of the cheek. Percussion or tapping of the tooth will provoke a painful response, but the tooth will not be sensitive to hot or cold applications. Contributing factors include calculus, foreign bodies, bacteria, and trauma.

Patient will complain of deep throbbing pain. The tooth will feel elevated in the socket, and the surrounding gingiva will be red, swollen, and tender.

Treatment

Attempt to drain the abscess through the gum crevice around the tooth by using a curette. Probe and locate any foreign bodies by spreading the tissue apart. Irrigate the pus and debris from the abscessed area. Advise the patient to rinse the mouth with hot saline solution every hour. For advanced cases that involve elevated temperature and general malaise, administer an antibiotic regimen and pain medication as needed.

ACUTE PERIAPICAL ABSCESS

Acute periapical abscess is an oral infection near the root end/apex/tip of the tooth and inflammation of the pulp. If the abscess is left untreated, the infection will spread to the surrounding space of the alveolar bone, periodontal ligament, deep structures of the neck, and the gingiva. The pus will accumulate, placing pressure on the tooth, which will be described by the patient as feeling "high." When the upper and lower teeth are brought together, the suspected tooth will feel like the first to impact the opposing tooth. Start percussion

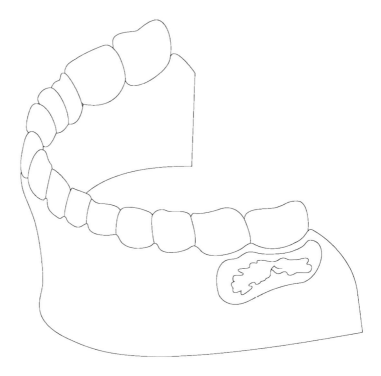

Acute periapical abscess—an infection near the root of the tooth.

from a normal tooth and continue to the suspected tooth. The suspected tooth will elicit a painful response from the patient. The gingival tissues will be tender and swollen around the area of the tooth.

Treatment

Treat the abscess aggressively to alleviate the patient's pain by opening the pulp chamber to allow for drainage. Make an incision with a #11 blade at the area over the maximum fluctuance. The incision is made through the gum and down to the bone. Place a drain using a section of a rubber band, cotton wick, section of surgical glove, or similar device that will facilitate drainage. Drainage of the site will usually provide relief from the pain. Severe cases of periapical abscess should be treated with antibiotic therapy, and extraction of the tooth should be considered as a last resort. Do not extract a suspected tooth until the patient has been adequately treated with antibiotic therapy. The bacteria will cascade into the patient's circulation from surgical manipulation and will place him or her at risk if not properly treated with antibiotic therapy for the infection.

ACUTE NECROTIZING ULCERATIVE GINGIVITIS

Acute necrotizing ulcerative gingivitis (trench mouth; Vincent's disease) is a bacterial infection that causes ulcers and tissue necrosis. The progression of the infection will involve the lips, cheeks, and facial bones. The patient will have foul odors of the mouth and will complain of a strong metallic taste. The gingiva will be inflamed and bleeding. The patient will have a constant gnawing pain, along with fever and general malaise. Contributing factors include poor oral hygiene, improper diet, alcohol use, tobacco use, suppressed immune system, previous infections, stress, and environmental factors.

Treatment
Advise the patient to rinse his or her mouth every hour with salt water and hydrogen peroxide solution for the next three days. Have the patient brush with a soft bristle toothbrush when he or she is able to tolerate the brushing and can continue with the regimen on an hourly basis. When the patient is able to tolerate brushing and flossing, he or she will then discontinue the hydrogen peroxide rinse and continue with brushing and flossing. Advise the patient to brush three times a day and floss at least once a day. A chlorhexidine (Peridex) rinse twice a day for the next five days can be incorporated into the regimen.

Educate the patient on proper oral hygiene for cleaning and scaling of the teeth. Advise on proper diet high in protein, vitamins, and fluid intake. Monitor the patient for continued tissue breakdown or systemic changes.

LUDWIG'S ANGINA

Ludwig's angina is a bacterial infection that involves primarily the sublingual and submaxillary space. The floor of the mouth, areas underneath the tongue, and the chin become inflamed and the tissues begin to swell. Typical causes of the infection are attributed to abscesses forming at the root of a tooth or trauma to the mouth. The swelling of the involved tissue can be life threatening by occluding the patient's airway. The patient will experience difficulty breathing, mental confusion, fever, neck pain, swelling around the neck, fatigue, and drooling.

Treatment
Airway first! If the patient's airway is compromised, intubation, surgical airway, or a cricothyrotomy is needed immediately to correct the airway obstruction. Antibiotic therapy should be administered as soon as possible with a broad-spectrum antibiotic. Incise and drain the abscess. Transport the patient to a medical facility for definitive care.

CAVERNOUS SINUS THROMBOSIS

The blood pressure of the cavernous sinus may be lower than the surrounding vessels. This causes the blood flow to reverse direction or back up and pool in the cavernous sinus. An infection from the sinuses, ears, or teeth moves against the venous blood flow and will cause an obstruction and deep space swelling. The venous obstruction causes paresis of the third, fourth, and sixth cranial nerve. The patient will present with bulging or drooping eyes, fatigue, loss of vision, limited movement of the eye, and increased body temperature and heart rate.

Treatment

Administer a broad-spectrum antibiotic. Transport the patient to a medical facility for definitive care.

FACIAL ABSCESS

Swelling can occur after a tooth has been extracted or during an infection. The swelling will involve the areas around the palate, sublingual, and eyes. The patient will complain of pain, fever, chills, and fatigue.

Treatment

For patients without suppuration: administer antibiotic therapy of Pen VK or Erythromycin.

For patients with suppuration: incise and drain abscess. Administer antibiotic therapy of Pen VK or Erythromycin.

DENTAL KITS

Dental tools are sold as individual pieces or as a complete set. For every expedition that requires dental care for extended periods, the individual medical practitioner/operator must consider the cost of the equipment and the weight that he or she must carry to the site.

The practitioner/operator's skill level is another important factor in determining the amount and type of dental tools to be carried into any remote and austere environment. The best dental tools are of no value if the practitioner/operator does not have the ability to use the tools with a high degree of proficiency.

Commercial dental kits provide a way to treat individuals with immediate first aid. They can be used by the layperson and do not require a high degree of dental proficiency. The more advanced kits will serve a wide variety of dental needs and require a better understanding of dental anatomy, injuries, treatment, and procedures.

Every dental kit, from basic to advanced, should address ways to manage pain and blood loss. Determine the quality of the tools needed based on mission profile, availability, weight, and special considerations. Do not overlook sterilization when metal dental tools will be used with multiple patients.

DENTAL FIRST-AID KIT

A dental first-aid kit can be purchased for a small fee from

Walmart, Walgreens, Rite Aid, or CVS. The items found in these kits are made of plastic and will not have the strength needed for repeated use on extended expeditions under difficult conditions. The kit will take up very little room in a field pack and should be revised for each outing. Small dental first-aid kits can be carried by any individual on an expedition or operation.

Tools
❏ dental mirror
❏ explorer or pick/cleaner
❏ small spatula
❏ cotton tip applicators
❏ 2 x 2 gauze
❏ gloves

Any or all of the following
❏ nontoxic super glue
❏ baby teething gel
❏ cavity varnish
❏ eugenol
❏ stomadhesive
❏ dental cement (zinc oxide)

Medications for minor pain management
❏ ibuprofen or acetaminophen

BASIC DENTAL KIT

The content of the basic dental kit is molded by the preference of the operator. The tools are sturdier and therefore heavier than plastic instruments. This should be taken into consideration for operations where all equipment will be carried in by the practitioner/operator.

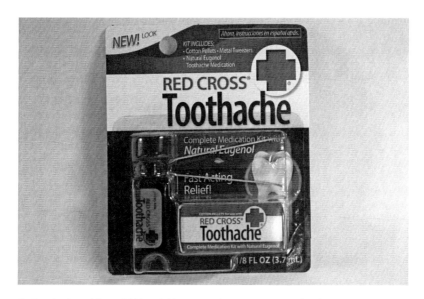

A simple dental first aid kit sold in stores for common toothaches.

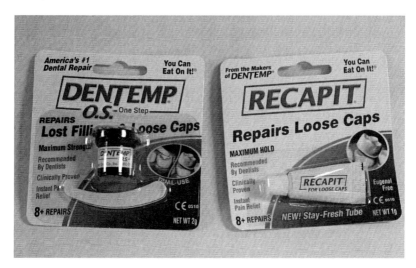

Two examples of dental first aid kits sold in stores for temporary fillings and emergencies.

Tools

- ❏ dental mirror
- ❏ #5 double-ended explorer/probe
- ❏ double-ended excavator
- ❏ elevator
- ❏ double-ended plug/filler
- ❏ #150 universal forceps upper and #151 universal forceps lower
- ❏ scalpel handle
- ❏ #11 and #15 blades
- ❏ scissors
- ❏ hemostat
- ❏ angle-point tweezers
- ❏ needle driver
- ❏ syringe for irrigation
- ❏ cotton tip applicators
- ❏ cotton balls
- ❏ gauze
- ❏ dental floss

Any or all of the following

- ❏ nontoxic super glue
- ❏ baby teething gel
- ❏ cavity varnish (Copalite)
- ❏ eugenol
- ❏ stomadhesive
- ❏ dental cement (zinc oxide)
- ❏ Cidex for cold sterilization in the absence of an autoclave

Anesthetic

- ❏ 2 percent lidocaine

Sutures

- ❏ operator's choice

DENTAL KITS

Any of the following hemostatic agents

❏ ActCel
❏ Celox
❏ similar product meant for the oral cavity

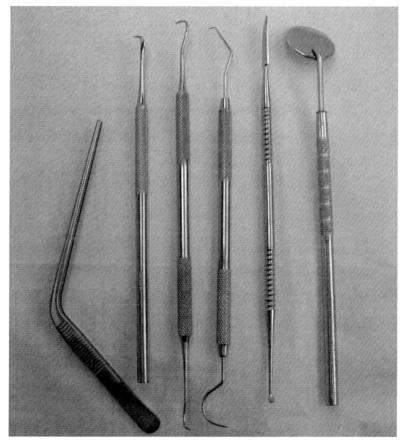

Common dental tools found in the standard operator's kit. From left to right: angle-point tweezer, a scaler, two different types of explorers/probes, a double-ended spatula/tamp, and a dental mirror.

ADVANCED DENTAL KIT

The content of the advanced dental kit is molded by the preference of the operator. Weight will be significant and will play a role when determining the risks/benefits to the operation.

Tools
❏ dental mirror
❏ #5 double-ended explorer/probe
❏ double-ended excavator
❏ elevator
❏ double-ended plug/filler
❏ #150 universal forceps upper and #151 universal forceps lower
❏ scalpel handle
❏ #11 and #15 blades
❏ scissors
❏ hemostat
❏ angle-point tweezers
❏ needle driver
❏ syringe for irrigation
❏ curette/scaler
❏ bone rongeur
❏ bone rasp
❏ cotton tip applicators
❏ cotton balls
❏ gauze
❏ dental floss
❏ portable handheld dental drill

All of the following
❏ nontoxic super glue
❏ baby teething gel

- ❑ cavity varnish (Copalite)
- ❑ eugenol
- ❑ stomadhesive
- ❑ dental cement (zinc oxide)
- ❑ Fuji IX ionomer
- ❑ Cidex for cold sterilization in the absence of an autoclave

Anesthetics
- ❑ 2 percent lidocaine
- ❑ 3 percent mepivacaine
- ❑ 5 percent bupivacaine

Sutures
- ❑ operator's choice

Any of the following hemostatic agents
- ❑ ActCel
- ❑ Celox
- ❑ similar product meant for the oral cavity